Beating

Cookbook

The Delicious & Healthy Recipes to Prevent & Combat Cancer

BY: Stephanie Sharp

Copyright © 2019 by Stephanie Sharp

License Notes

Copyright 2020 by Stephanie Sharp All rights reserved.

No part of this Book may be transmitted or reproduced into any format for any means without the proper permission of the Author. This includes electronic or mechanical methods, photocopying or printing.

The Reader assumes all risk when following any of the guidelines or ideas written as they are purely suggestion and for informational purposes. The Author has taken every precaution to ensure accuracy of the work but bears no responsibility if damages occur due to a misinterpretation of suggestions.

wwwwwwwwwwwwwwwwwwwwwwww

Table of Contents

Introduction 6

Cinnamon Apple Quinoa 8

Almond Pancakes with Strawberry Puree 10

Scrambled Tofu Garlic 12

Apple and Beet Salads 14

Smooth Avocado Toast 16

Mashed Sweet Potatoes 18

Blueberry Muesli 20

Apple and Carrot Muffin 22

Baked Beans in Toast 25

Oats Cinnamon Waffle 27

Avocado Veggie Salads 29

Quinoa and Beans Patties 31

Braised Garlic Kale 34

Stuffed Eggplants 36

Stir Fry Tofu Broccoli 38

Wheat Tortilla Lettuce 40

Artichoke Pizza with Chickpeas Dough......................... 42

Healthy Cauliflower Rice.. 45

Chicken Lettuce Salads 47

Broccoli Clear Soup 49

Stuffed Artichoke with Cauliflower Rice...................... 51

Creamy Carrot Soup... 55

Tamarind Fresh Mackerel 58

Strawberry Apple Chicken 61

Roasted Tofu with Sesame Seeds.................................... 64

Sautéed Carrots 67

Original Roasted Pumpkin 69

Brown Eggplant Black Pepper 71

Green Spinach Fritter 73

Coconut Ginger Muffins 75

Conclusion 77

About the Author 78

Author's Afterthoughts 79

Introduction

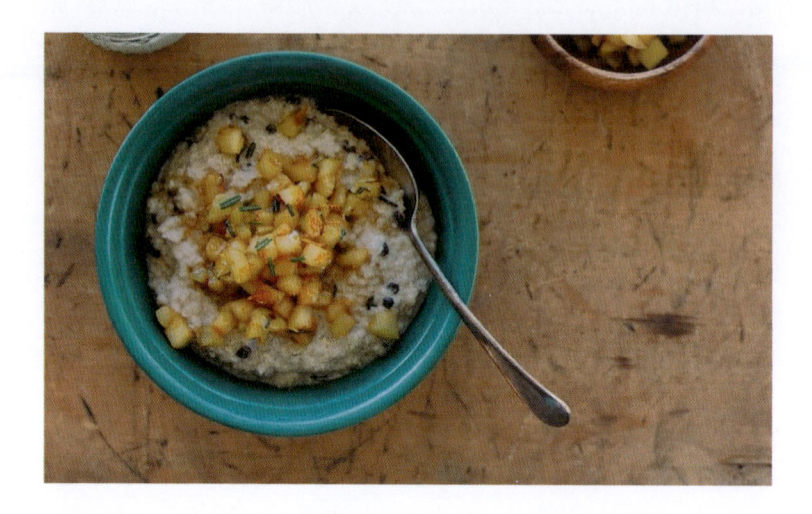

Healthy food choices are crucial in the daily eating habits of cancer patients, more so, for those persons who want to prevent their bodies from getting cancer. Having a healthier lifestyle combined with good eating habits will limit the risk of having cancer and more people who have suffered from it can be saved.

Cancer Cookbook provides 30 healthy recipes that are beneficial in the prevention of cancer and helping to beat it. With these recipes, this book will help you to create healthy meal plans for your loved ones and you. The recipes listed are geared to help you plan your diet properly and have a healthier lifestyle. The short description associated with each recipe will make it easier for you to imagine and serve the most appropriate and enticing food on your dining table.

Get your copy of this book today and start enjoying a healthier eating lifestyle.

Cinnamon Apple Quinoa

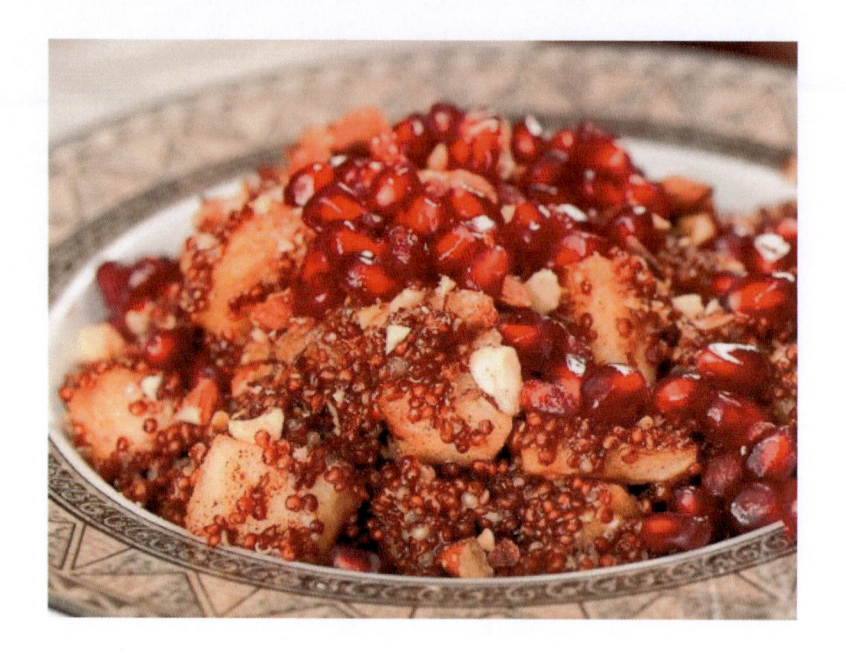

Known as an ancient beneficial grain, quinoa is a good food to combat cancer. Having quinoa as breakfast is really a great choice to start the day.

Serves: 2

Time: 30 mins.

Ingredients:

- 1-cup quinoa
- 4 cups water
- 1-cup oatmeal
- 2 tablespoons raw honey
- 1-teaspoon cinnamon
- ½ cup apple wedge

Directions:

1. Pour water into a large pot then brings to boil.

2. Once it is boiled, add the quinoa and oatmeal into the pot then stirs well.

3. Reduce the heat then cooks until the water is completely absorbed into the quinoa.

4. Remove from the heat then quickly stir in honey and cinnamon. Mix well.

5. Put on a serving dish then top with apple wedges. Serve and enjoy right away.

Almond Pancakes with Strawberry Puree

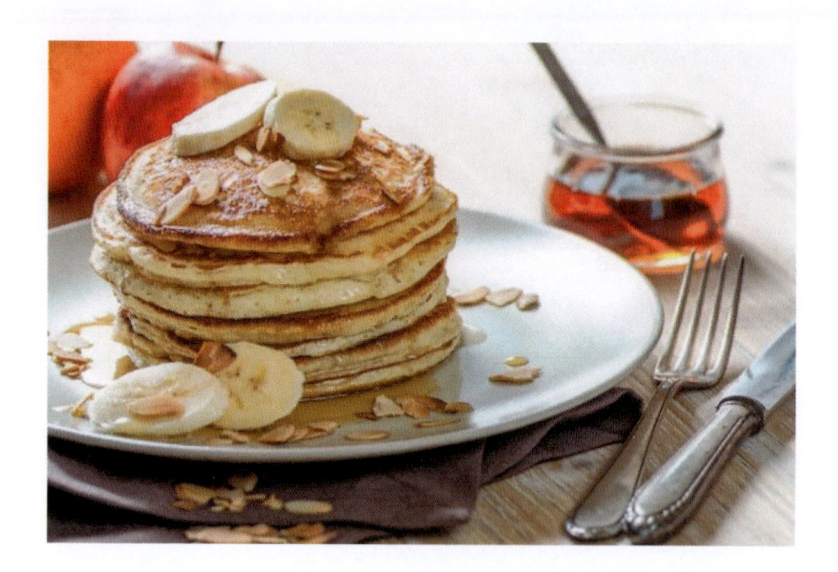

This breakfast menu is very light and soft. This breakfast is rich of nutrients that will function as a fuel for your busy day. As the topping, strawberry puree will serve as a taste enhancer as its sour flavor and chunky texture is so contrast with the taste and texture of the pancake. For variation, you can substitute the strawberry with some other kinds of berries or fruits of your preference.

Serves: 4

Time: 15 mins.

Ingredients:

- 1 ½ cups almond flour
- 1 cup almond milk
- 2 tablespoons honey
- 1-teaspoon olive oil
- 1-cup fresh strawberries

Directions:

1. Set aside your olive oil and fresh strawberry then combine all the remaining ingredients in a bowl.

2. Whisk the ingredients until incorporated and smooth.

3. Preheat a pan over medium heat then coat with olive oil.

4. Once it is hot, pour about 3 tablespoons of mixture into the pan then cooks and flips until the pancake is lightly golden.

5. Transfer the pancake to a serving dish then repeat with the remaining ingredients.

6. Just before serving, place all of the strawberries in a food processor. Process until smooth.

7. Pour the smooth strawberry over the pancakes then serve immediately.

Scrambled Tofu Garlic

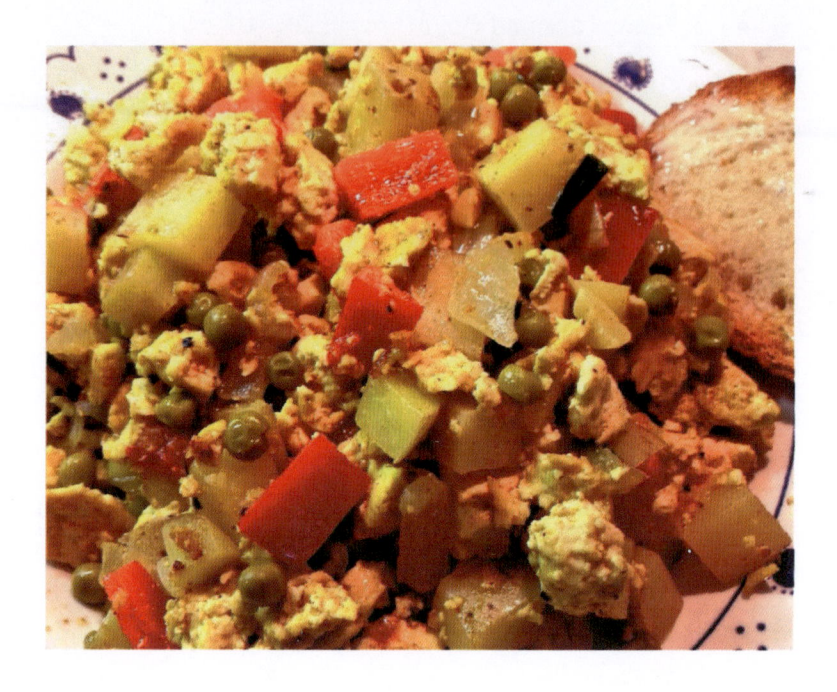

This kind of protein is good to prevent and fight cancer compare to animal protein like meat because it will not trigger the development and the spreading of the cancer cells. Another advantage of this recipe is it is so easy to prepare and take a very short time to cook.

Serves: 4

Time: 10 mins.

Ingredients:

- ½ lb. firm tofu
- 2 teaspoons olive oil
- 2 teaspoons minced garlic
- ½ teaspoon pepper

Directions:

1. Cut the tofu into small cubes then set aside.

2. Preheat a skillet over medium heat then pours olive oil into the skillet.

3. Once it is hot, stir in minced garlic then sautés until lightly golden and aromatic.

4. Add tofu into the skillet then quickly stirs and chops the tofu until becoming scrambles.

5. Season with pepper then transfers to a serving dish. Serve and enjoy.

Apple and Beet Salads

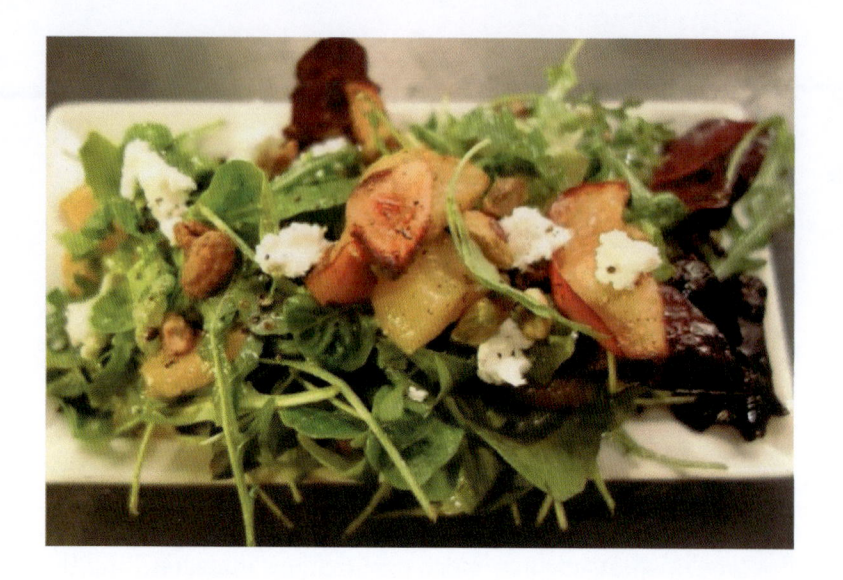

The first thing that is suitable to describe this breakfast menu is that it is totally healthy. Beet is known for its function as an antioxidant agent. On the other hand, apple is also famous for its many health benefits. The combination of the two popular healthy fruits is perfect to treat or prevent cancer, as it will boost the growth of new cells and improve your stamina.

Serves: 4

Time: 15 mins.

Ingredients:

- 1 cup shredded apple
- 1 cup shredded beet
- ½ cup fresh orange juice
- 1 teaspoon minced garlic
- 4 tablespoons olive oil
- ¼ teaspoon pepper

Directions:

1. Place minced garlic and pepper in a bowl then pours olive oil and orange juice into the bowl. Stir well.

2. Add shredded apple and beet into the bowl then toss to combine.

3. Let the salad sit for 30 minutes, you can chill it in the refrigerator.

4. Remove from the refrigerator after 30 minutes then enjoy right away.

Smooth Avocado Toast

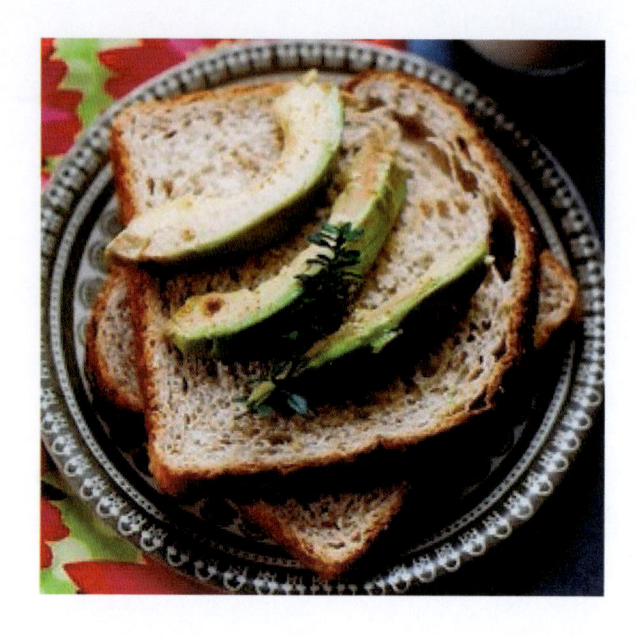

Another healthy choice of plant-based fat and protein is avocado. The kind of protein inside the fruit is relatively easier to be absorbed by the body. It is also healthier compare to the animal-based fat. This avocado spread also taste really well. It is also best to sprinkle the spread with some almond or chestnuts.

Serves: 2

Time: 15 mins.

Ingredients:

- 1 ripe avocado
- 2 slices whole grain bread
- ½ teaspoon cinnamon
- 2 teaspoons honey

Directions:

1. Toast the whole grain breads then place on a serving dish.

2. Cut the avocado into halves then discards the seed.

3. Scoop out the avocado flesh then mash until smooth.

4. Spread the smooth avocado over the toast the sprinkles cinnamon over the avocado.

5. Drizzle honey on top then serves. Enjoy immediately.

Mashed Sweet Potatoes

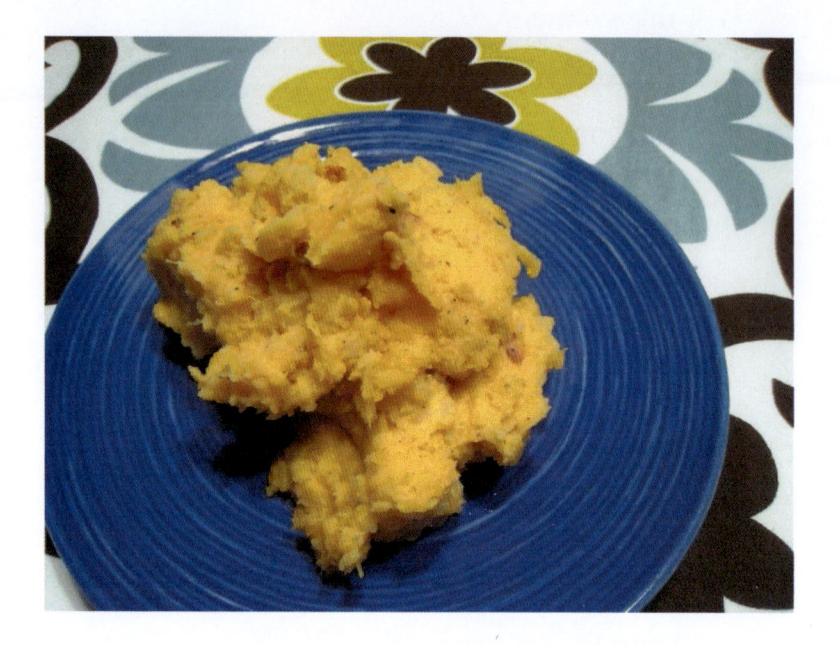

One great advantage of consuming this food is that it can satisfy your appetite although it is served in small portion. Sweet potatoes provide healthy source of carbs because it contains natural glucose that can be absorb easily by our body.

Serves: 2

Time: 15 mins.

Ingredients:

- 1 lb. sweet potatoes
- 2 tablespoons coconut milk
- 2 tablespoons honey
- ½ teaspoon black pepper
- ¼ teaspoon cinnamon ¼ teaspoon nutmeg

Directions:

1. Preheat an oven to 400°F then lines a baking sheet with parchment paper.

2. Using a fork prick the sweet potatoes several times then place on the prepared baking pan.

3. Bake for 30 minutes or until the sweet potatoes are tender.

4. Once it is done, remove from the oven then let them warm.

5. Peel the cooked sweet potatoes then using a potato masher mash then sweet potatoes until smooth.

6. Add the remaining ingredients into the smooth sweet potato then mix well. Serve and enjoy right away.

Blueberry Muesli

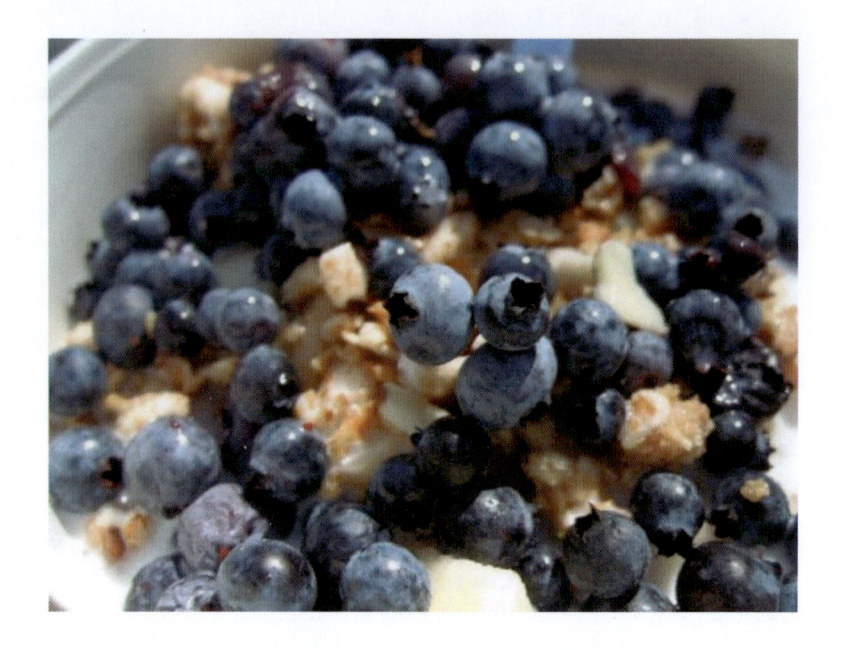

If you wish to eat something light in the morning, this is a perfect choice. This food is great for cancer patients because of the ingredients chosen for this recipe. Oats and blueberry are just a touch of freshness and energy source for your busy day. Add some nuts or other fruits in the list that you like if you want some variations.

Serves: 2

Time: 15 mins.

Ingredients:

- ¾ cup rolled oats
- 4 tablespoons walnuts
- 1-teaspoon cinnamon
- 1-cup fresh blueberries
- 1-cup fresh orange juice

Directions:

1. Preheat an oven to 325°F then lines a baking sheet with parchment paper.

2. Place oats, walnuts, and cinnamon in a bowl then mix well.

3. Spread on your prepared baking sheet then bake for 10 minutes. Stirring occasionally.

4. Remove from the oven then let it cool for a few minutes.

5. Transfer to a serving bowl then sprinkles with fresh blueberries. Serve the muesli with fresh orange juice. Enjoy!

Apple and Carrot Muffin

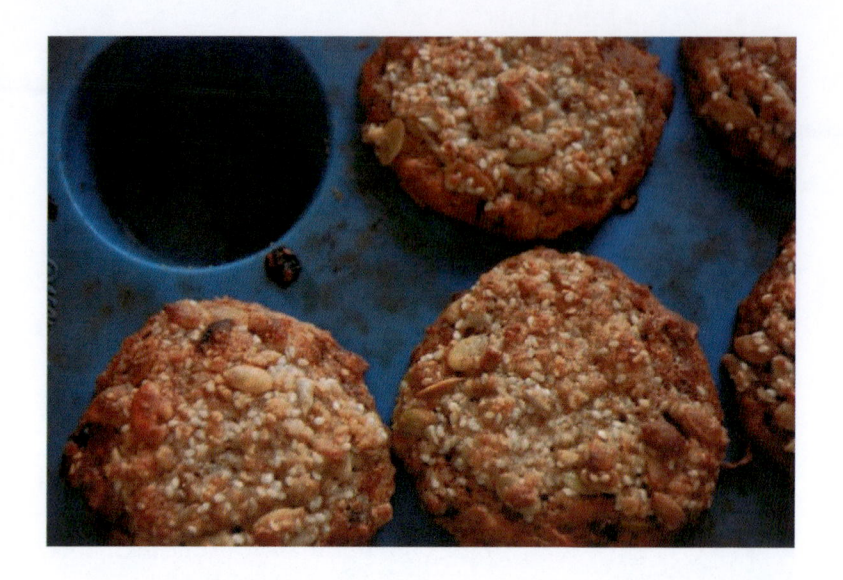

Grab this breakfast choice if you have a busy day. Some people will feel reluctant to eat when they are sick, but you can be sure that this muffin is an excellent choice of a rich of an antioxidant recipe.

Serves: 4

Time: 25 mins.

Ingredients:

- ½ cups grated carrot
- ½ cup grated apple2 organic eggs
- 4 tablespoons coconut milk
- 3 tablespoons raw honey
- 1-teaspoon ginger
- 1 cup almond flour
- 1-teaspoon cinnamon
- ¼ teaspoon nutmeg

Directions:

1. Preheat an oven to 375°F then coat 8 muffin cups. Set aside.

2. Crack the eggs then place in a bowl.

3. Add ginger and honey then pours coconut milk into the bowl. Mix well.

4. Stir in grated carrot and apple into the mixture then add almond flour together with cinnamon and nutmeg. Mix to combine.

5. Divide the mixture into the prepared muffin cups then bake for 20 minutes.

6. Once it is done, remove from the oven and enjoy.

Baked Beans in Toast

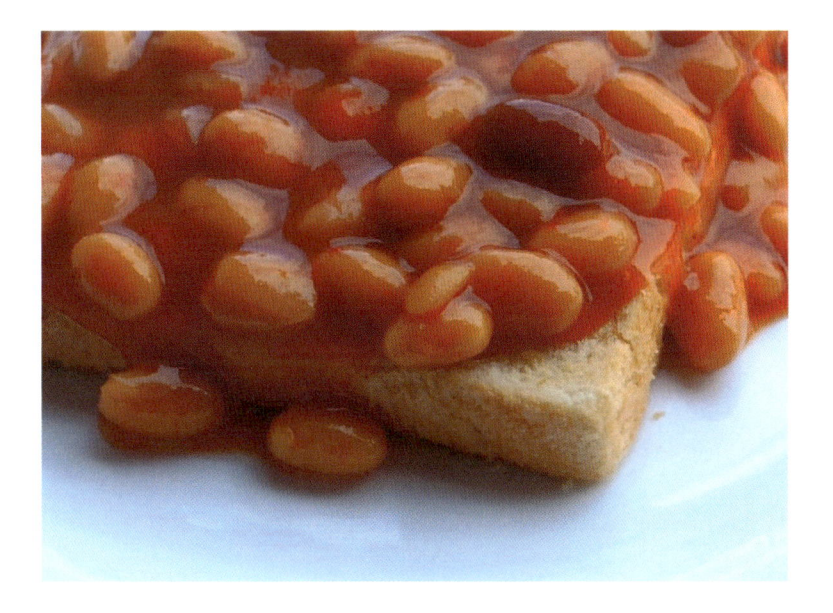

By looking at its appearance, you must agree that this is a delicious snack you cannot resist. The combination of the beans and the spices are so mouthwatering. Beans are also a good food for cancer treatment and prevention as it has phytosterols that is proven to reduce the risk of cancer.

Serves: 2

Time: 20 mins.

Ingredients:

- 1 cup cooked beans
- 2 teaspoons olive oil
- 1 teaspoon minced garlic
- 2 tablespoons tomato puree
- 1-teaspoon paprika
- 2 slices wholegrain bread
- ½ teaspoon black pepper

Directions:

1. Preheat a skillet over medium heat then pours olive oil into it.

2. Stir in minced garlic then sautés until lightly brown and aromatic.

3. Add tomato puree and paprika into the skillet then bring to boil.

4. Once it is boiled, stir in cooked beans then bring to a simmer.

5. Meanwhile, toast the whole grain bread then place on a serving dish.

6. Spread the beans over the bread then sprinkle pepper on top. Serve and enjoy warm.

Oats Cinnamon Waffle

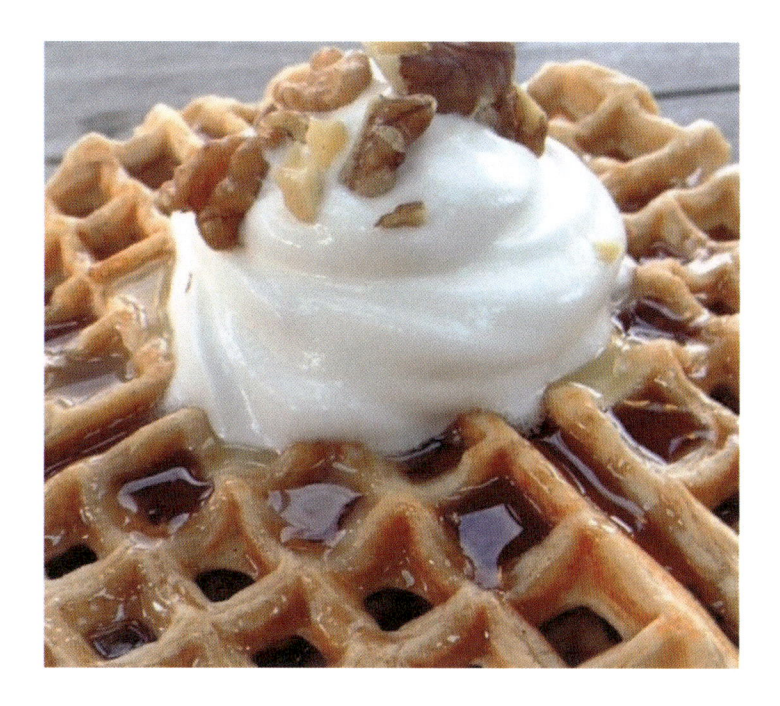

What is easier to prepare for breakfast than waffle? To create a friendly-food for cancer patient, oats are added as the basic ingredient. Pour some honey for better taste.

Serves: 4

Time: 15 mins.

Ingredients:

- ½ cup rolled oats
- 2 cups almond milk
- ½ cups almond flour
- 1-teaspoon cinnamon
- 2 tablespoons raw honey

Directions:

1. Add all your ingredients in a blender then blend until smooth and incorporated.

2. Preheat a waffle cast iron over medium heat then cook the waffle according to the machine instructions.

3. Transfer waffles to a serving dish then enjoy warm.

Avocado Veggie Salads

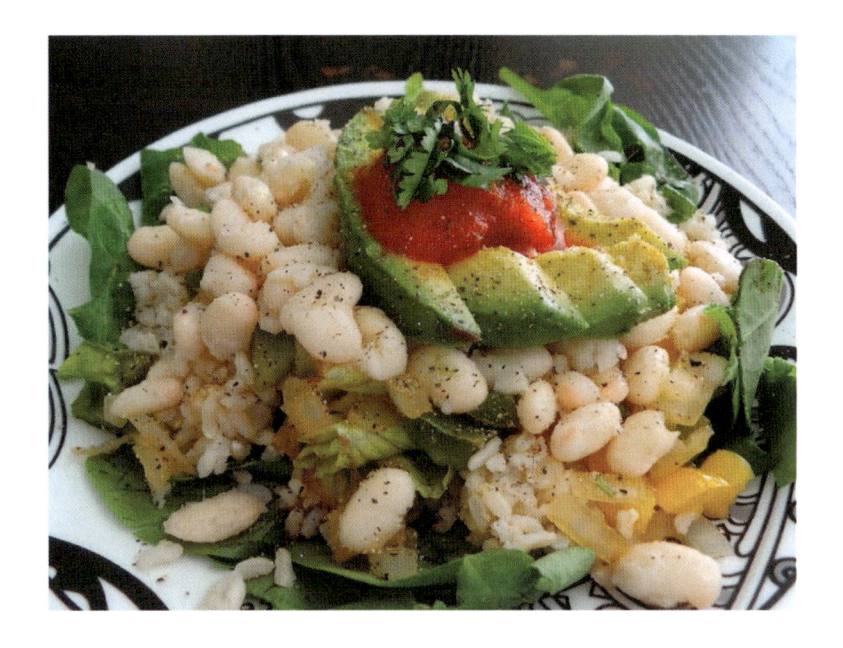

As stated earlier, avocado is a good choice of food for cancer prevention and cure because of some reasons. You can serve avocado in many different ways. One of the best avocado recipes is to make it as salads. With some mixture of other green and orange vegetables, this avocado veggie salad is a healthy afternoon treat.

Serves: 4

Time: 15 mins.

Ingredients:

- 2 medium ripe tomatoes
- 1 ripe avocado
- 1 cup chopped lettuce
- 2 tablespoons chopped onion
- 3 teaspoons olive oil
- 2 teaspoons lemon juice
- ¼ teaspoon pepper

Directions:

1. Cut the tomato into slices then place in a salad bowl.

2. Peel the avocado then cut into wedges. Discard the seed.

3. Place the avocado in the same salad bowl with the tomato then drizzle olive oil and lemon juice over the salads.

4. Sprinkle pepper on top then toss to combine.

5. Arrange the lettuce on a serving dish then transfer the salads on top.

6. Enjoy right away or chill in the refrigerator if you want to consume it later.

Quinoa and Beans Patties

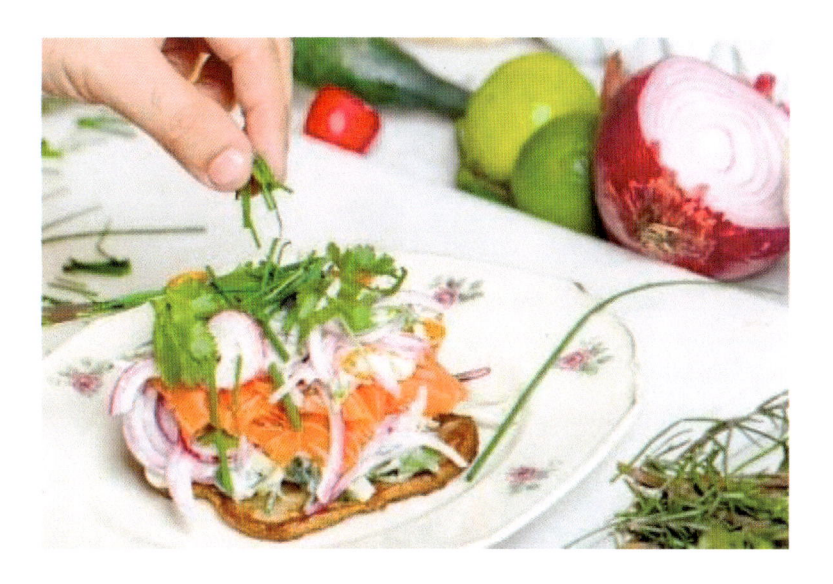

Pork or meat patties may not be a great choice of food to fight cancer. As an alternative, quinoa and beans patties can be delicious and tasty lunch menu. To enhance the flavor, you can serve it with avocado dip or other sauce of your preferences.

Serves: 4

Time: 25 mins.

Ingredients:

- ¾ cup cooked organic black beans
- 4 tablespoons quinoa
- ½ cup fresh water
- ½ cup diced bell pepper
- 2 tablespoons chopped onion
- 2 teaspoons minced garlic
- 1-teaspoon cumin
- ½ cup mashed sweet potatoes
- 2 tablespoons olive oil

Directions:

1. Pour water into a saucepan then add quinoa into the saucepan. Bring to boil.

2. Once it is boiled, reduce the heat then bring to a simmer until the water has completely absorbed into the quinoa.

3. Transfer the cooked quinoa to a food processor then add cooked black beans, mashed potato, and bell pepper into the food processor.

4. Season with chopped onion, minced garlic, and cumin then process until smooth.

5. Shape the mixture into medium patty form then let it sit for a few minutes.

6. Meanwhile, preheat a pan over medium heat then pour olive oil into it.

7. Add the patties to the pan the fry until both sides of the patties are lightly golden.

8. Arrange the patties on a serving dish then enjoy warm.

Braised Garlic Kale

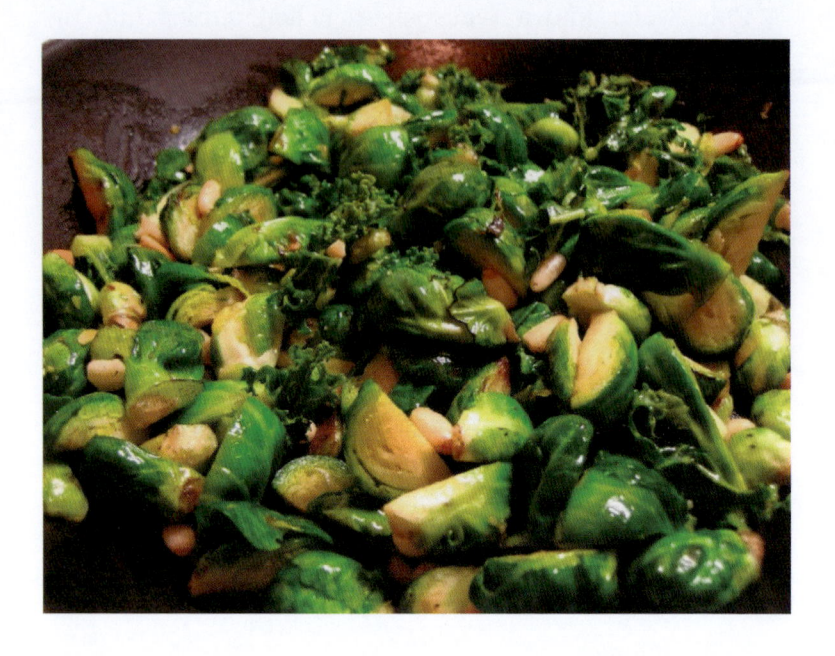

Kale is a miraculous vegetable since these green leaves contain a lot of vitamins and minerals. Nutritionists even call it as the richest nutrient food on earth. Therefore, I suggest this as the best food for cancer cure and prevention.

Serves: 4

Time: 10 mins.

Ingredients:

- 2 cups chopped kale
- 2 teaspoons olive oil
- 3 teaspoons minced garlic
- ½ cup water
- ¼ teaspoon pepper

Directions:

1. Preheat skillet over medium heat then pour olive oil into it.

2. Stir in minced garlic then sautés until lightly golden and aromatic.

3. Add chopped kale to the skillet then pours water into the skillet.

4. Season with pepper then cook until the kale is wilted.

5. Transfer to a serving dish then enjoys right away.

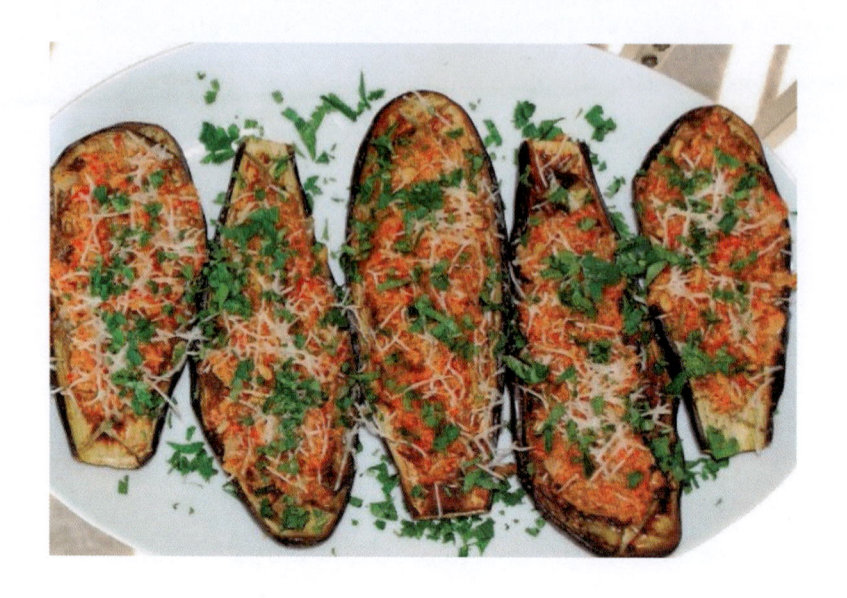

Stuffed Eggplants

Eggplants, especially the one planted organically, is one food that is highly recommended for cancer patients. It is full of nutrients that can help your cell regeneration and improve immune systems. Some of the nutrients inside the eggplants include vitamin C, nasunin and chlorogenic antioxidant agents, and magnesium. It is also a kind of food to prevent cancer as the content of the eggplants can help your body to fight the free radicals that trigger cancer.

Serves: 4

Time: 45 mins.

Ingredients:

- 4 eggplants
- 4 tablespoons olive oil
- ½ cup chopped onion
- 2 teaspoons minced garlic
- 2 tablespoons diced tomato
- 1 cup chopped carrots
- 1 cup chopped pepper
- ½ teaspoon cumin
- ½ teaspoon black pepper

Directions:

1. Preheat an oven to 400 °F then lines a baking sheet with parchment paper.

2. Horizontally cut the eggplants into halves then arrange on the prepared baking sheet.

3. Combine diced tomato, carrots, and bell pepper then season with pepper, garlic, cumin, and onion.

4. Top each halved eggplant with the tomato mixture then bake for about 45 minutes or until done.

5. Remove from the oven then serves warm. Enjoy!

Stir Fry Tofu Broccoli

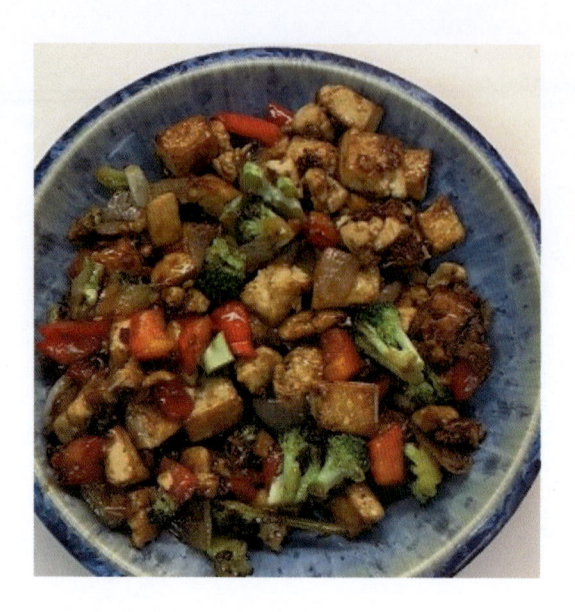

The benefits of tofu to fight cancer have been discussed earlier in the previous recipes. When the benefits of tofu are combined with the benefits of broccoli, they can serve as more powerful weapons to eradicate the cancer cells. Cell regeneration phase will speed up and your body will be in a better condition day by day if you consume it regularly.

Serves: 4

Time: 10 mins.

Ingredients:

- 1 lb. firm tofu
- 2 cups broccoli florets
- 2 teaspoons minced garlic
- 1 teaspoon red chili flakes
- 2 teaspoons olive oil

Directions:

1. Preheat skillet over the medium heat and then pour olive oil into it.

2. Stir in the minced garlic then sautés until lightly golden.

3. Add tofu, broccoli, and red chili flakes into the skillet then cook for a few minutes.

4. Once it is done, transfer to a serving dish then serves immediately.

Wheat Tortilla Lettuce

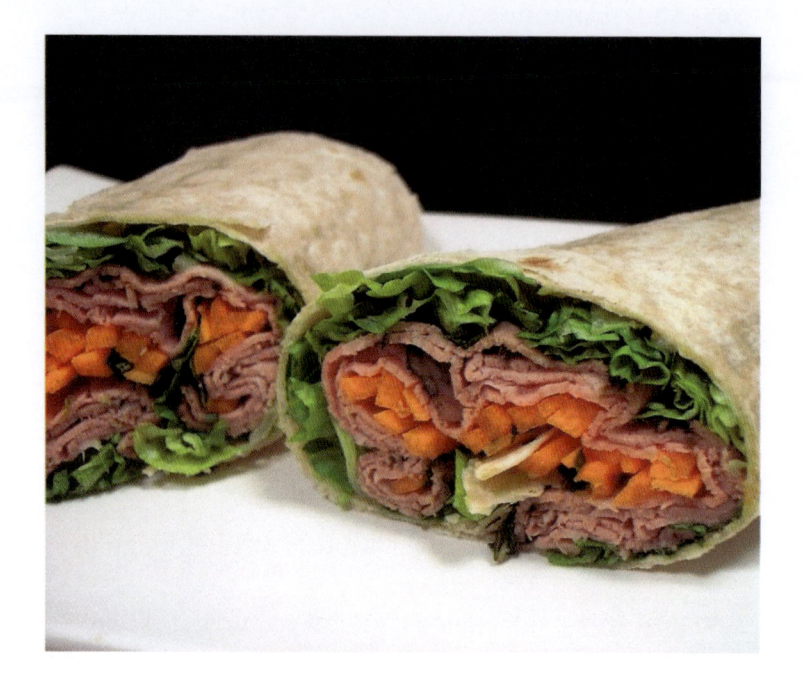

Take some bite to recharge your energy in the afternoon. This tortilla recipe is easy to make and healthy. Lettuce is known for its many benefits as what other green vegetables serve. Adding some slices of avocado or kale is also great.

Serves: 2

Time: 10 mins.

Ingredients:

- 1 cup chopped lettuce
- 1-teaspoon extra virgin olive oil
- 2 tablespoons chopped onion
- 2 whole-wheat tortillas

Directions:

1. Set your skillet to preheat over medium heat then pour olive oil into it.

2. Stir in onion and chopped lettuce then sauté until wilted.

3. Lay the tortillas flat then top with the sautéed lettuce.

4. Roll each tortilla then place on a serving dish. Serve and enjoy immediately.

Artichoke Pizza with Chickpeas Dough

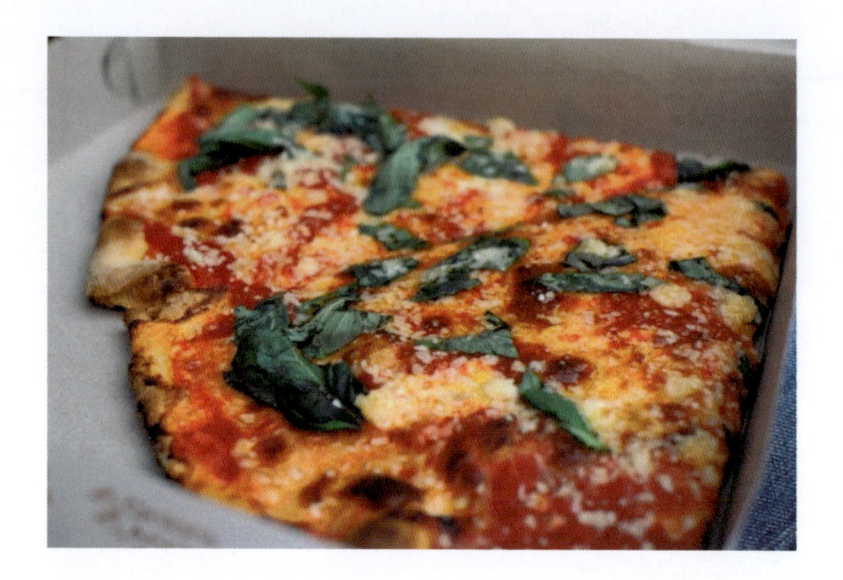

Buying a pan of pizza from a fast food restaurant is a big NO if you have cancer or want to prevent the disease. However, with this chickpea dough and artichoke topping, eating delicious pizza is possible. Both are known as two sources of food that are advisable for cancer patients.

Serves: 4

Time: 50 mins.

Ingredients:

- ¾ cup chickpea flour
- 1-cup water
- 1 ½ tablespoons olive oil

Topping:

- ½ cup mashed tomato
- ½ cup chopped cooked artichoke
- 2 tablespoons grated vegan cheese

Directions:

1. Preheat an oven to 350°F then coats a small pizza pan with cooking spray. Set aside.

2. Place chickpea flour in a bowl then pour olive oil and water into the bowl. Knead until becoming dough.

3. Transfer the mixture to the prepared pizza pan then spreads evenly and press.

4. For 25 minutes, Bake the crust until the top of the pizza crust is lightly golden.

5. Once it is done, take the crust out from the oven.

6. Quickly spread mashed tomato over the crust. Chop the artichoke then arrange on the crust.

7. Sprinkles grated vegan cheese on top then baked for 15 minutes.

8. Remove from the oven then let the pizza warm for a few minutes. Cut the pizza into wedges then serve warm.

Healthy Cauliflower Rice

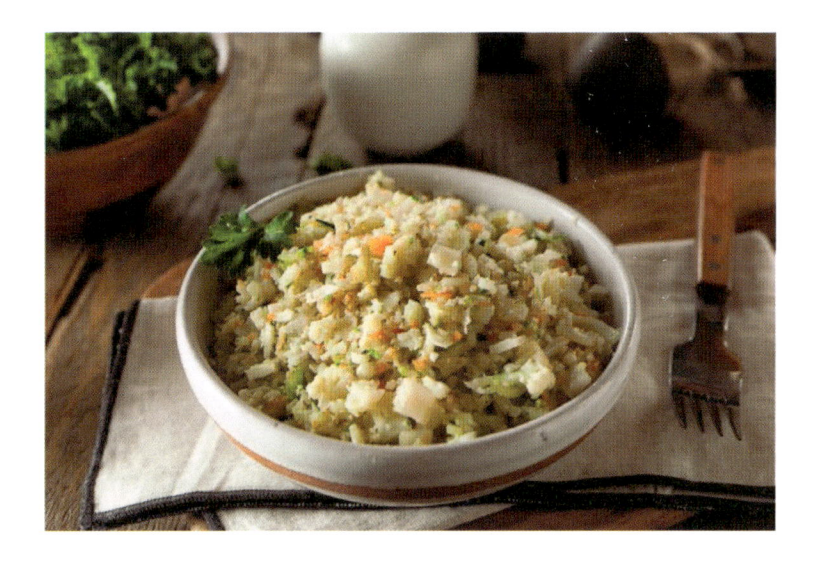

Sulforaphane consists in the cauliflower is scientifically proven to combat cancer cells. Therefore, even when you have already had cancer in your body, you can control its spreading as cauliflower can attack the cancer stem cell.

Serves: 4

Time: 15 mins.

Ingredients:

- 2 cups cauliflower florets
- ¼ cup olive oil
- ½ cup chopped onion
- 2 tablespoons lemon juice
- ½ teaspoon pepper
- 2 tablespoons chopped leek

Directions:

1. Preheat skillet over medium heat then pour olive oil into it.

2. Stir in chopped onion then sautés until translucent and aromatic.

3. Add cauliflower florets to the skillet then season with pepper.

4. Drizzle lemon juice over the cauliflower then sprinkles chopped leek on top. Cook the cauliflower until crispy.

5. Move the cooked cauliflower to a food processor the process until becoming crumbles. Serve and enjoy warm.

Chicken Lettuce Salads

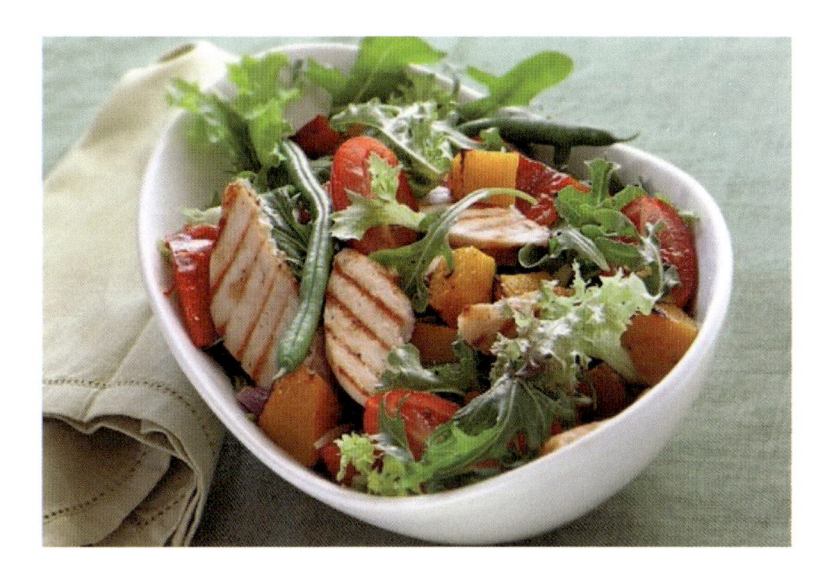

This is a selection recipe that is not only healthy but also so delicious, even for non-cancer patients. White meat is still appropriate to be consumed by cancer patients. Yet, it is important to choose the chicken from organic farms for a healthier choice.

Serves: 4

Time: 20 mins.

Ingredients:

- 1 lb. organic chicken breast
- ¼ cup olive oil
- 1-teaspoon thyme
- ½ teaspoon black pepper
- 3 cups chopped lettuce
- ¼ cup lemon juice

Directions:

1. Preheat a grill over medium heat.

2. Combine thyme with black pepper then add olive oil into the mixture. Stir well.

3. Use the spice mix to rub the chicken then grill the chicken until done.

4. Cut the chicken into slices then place in a salad bowl.

5. Add chopped lettuce into the bowl then drizzles lemon juice on top. toss to combine. Serve and enjoy right away.

Broccoli Clear Soup

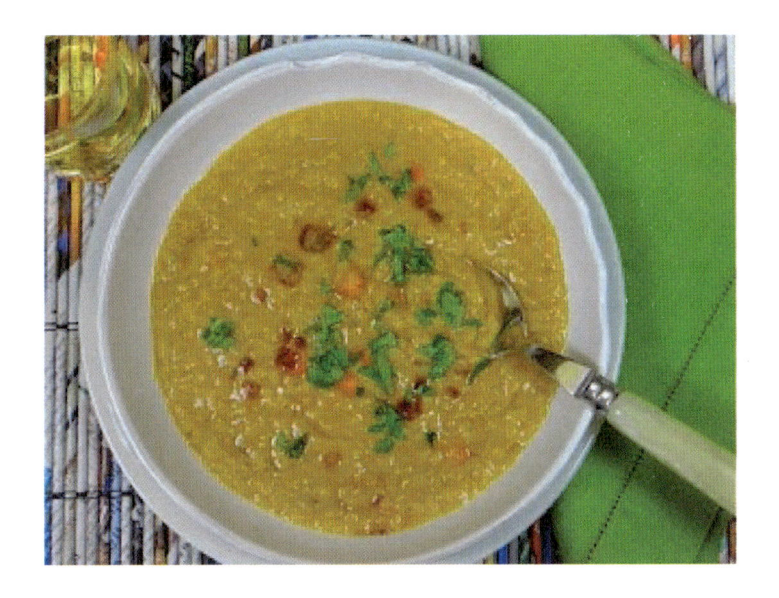

You know already the benefits of broccoli to eliminate cancer from the explanation provided in one of the previous recipes. One common mistake that common people do is to add thick creams and dairy products in the soup. Therefore, this clear soup is suggested as an option to a heavy cream soup.

Serves: 4

Time: 15 mins.

Ingredients:

- 1 lb. broccoli florets
- ¾ cup chopped onion
- 2 teaspoons minced garlic
- 4 cups low sodium vegetable broth
- 1 tablespoon chopped basil
- 2 tablespoons chopped parsley
- ½ teaspoon pepper

Directions:

1. Pour about a cup of vegetable broth in a pot then add garlic, chopped onion, pepper, and basil into the pot. Bring to boil.

2. Once it is boiled, stir in broccoli then pour the remaining broth into the pot. Bring to boil again.

3. Once it is boiled, reduce the heat and cook for about 5 minutes or until the broccoli is tender.

4. Transfer to a soup bowl then sprinkles chopped parsley on top. Serve and enjoy immediately.

Stuffed Artichoke with Cauliflower Rice

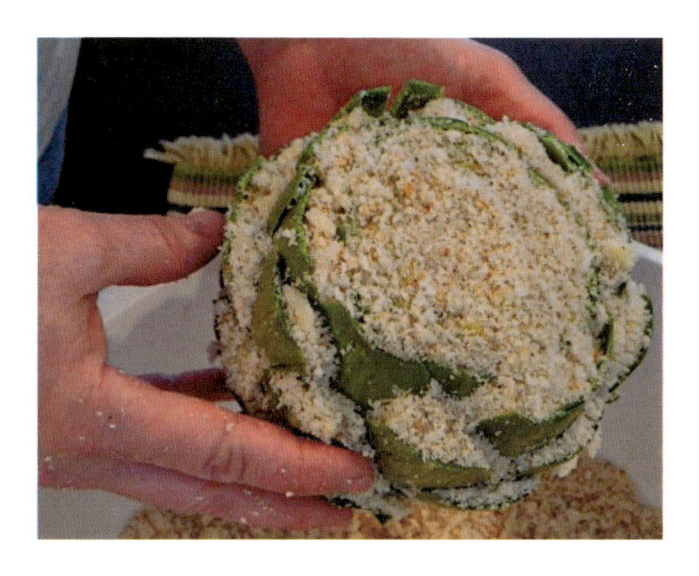

When the benefits of artichoke and cauliflower are combined, you will have countless reason to include this recipe in order to prevent yourself from cancer. This is also a good option if you are undergoing cancer treatment.

Serves: 4

Time: 25 mins.

Ingredients:

- 4 medium artichokes
- ½ cup cauliflower rice
- 2 teaspoons olive oil
- 1 tablespoon chopped celery
- 2 teaspoons minced garlic
- 4 tablespoons low sodium vegetable broth
- 2 tablespoons lemon

Directions:

1. Cut off the artichoke's stems and trim the outer leaves of the artichokes.

2. Chop the top of the artichokes so the top of the artichokes will be flat.

3. Pour water into a pot then add lemon juice in it. Bring to boil.

4. Once it is boiled, add the artichokes into the pot and cook for 15 minutes.

5. Remove the cooked artichokes from the water then set aside.

6. Next, preheat saucepan over medium heat then pour olive oil into it.

7. Stir in minced garlic then sautés until wilted and aromatic.

8. Pour vegetable broth into the saucepan then stir in cauliflower rice. Cook until the broth is completely absorbed into the cauliflower.

9. Sprinkle chopped celeries over the cauliflower rice then mix well.

10. Fill the artichokes with the cauliflower rice then using the back of a spoon, press until firm.

11. Arrange the artichokes on a serving dish then enjoy!

Creamy Carrot Soup

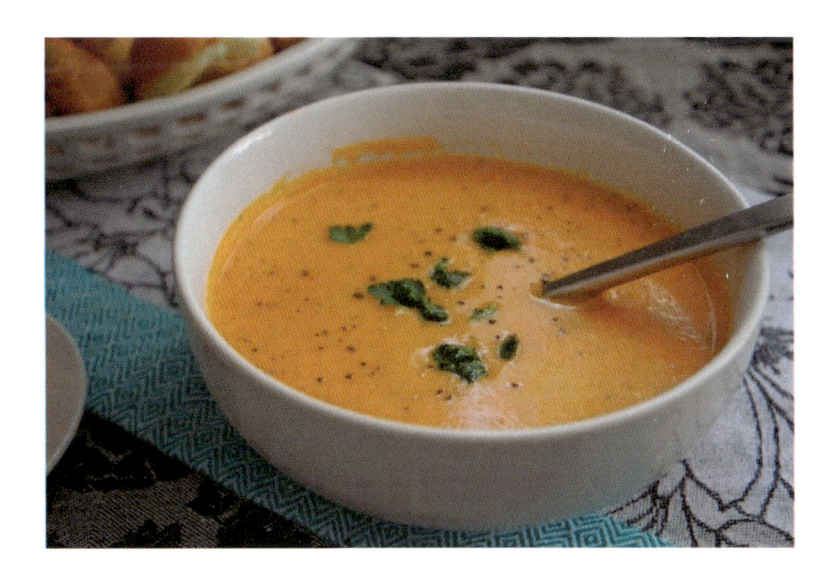

It is not a myth to say that orange fruits and vegetables are good to prevent or even cure cancer. It has been explained previously that those kinds of fruits and vegetables, such as pumpkins, tomatoes, and carrots are full of components that are beneficial for cancer treatment.

Serves: 4

Time: 25 mins.

Ingredients:

- 3 lbs. organic carrots
- 2 tablespoons olive oil
- 2 cups chopped onion
- 1-teaspoon ginger
- ¼ teaspoon cumin
- ¼ teaspoon cinnamon
- ¼ teaspoon turmeric
- ¼ teaspoon pepper
- 6 cups low sodium vegetable broth

Directions:

1. Preheat a saucepan then pour olive oil into it.

2. Once it is hot, stir in chopped onion then sautés until wilted and aromatic.

3. Transfer the sautéed onion to a pot then pour vegetable broth into it.

4. Cut the carrots into thick slices—you don't need to peel them, and then add into the pot.

5. Next, set your saucepan to preheat on medium heat then pour olive oil into it.

6. Once it is boiled, reduces the heat then cook the soup until the carrots are tender.

7. When the carrots are already tender, remove from heat and let the soup warm for a few minutes.

8. Using immersion blender, blend the soup until smooth and creamy.

9. Transfer the soup to the serving bowls then enjoy warm.

Tamarind Fresh Mackerel

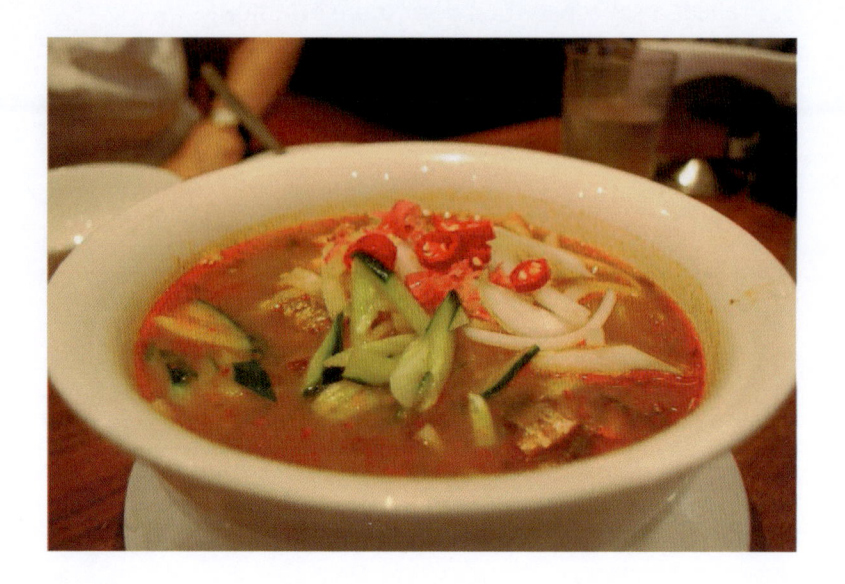

When it comes to animal-based protein, it is highly recommended to find either organic or non-pollutant habitat animals. If you are cancer patients, it is always important to know where your animal protein comes from and treated. Therefore, eating homemade food is the best option.

Serves: 3

Time: 25 mins.

Ingredients:

- 3 medium fresh mackerels
- 3 tablespoons olive oil
- 3 tablespoons minced garlic
- 3 tablespoons tamarind paste
- 3 tablespoons dill
- 1-tablespoon ginger
- ½ teaspoon cayenne pepper
- ½ teaspoon cumin
- 1-teaspoon coriander

Directions:

1. Set your oven to preheat to 350°F then lines a baking pan with aluminum foil. Set aside.

2. Place coriander, cumin, ginger, tamarind paste, and minced garlic in a bowl.

3. Pour olive oil into the spice mixture then mix well.

4. Using a sharp knife slash each mackerel then rub with the spice.

5. Arrange the mackerel on the prepared baking pan then sprinkle dill on top.

6. Bake for 25 minutes until the mackerels are completely cooked.

7. Once it is done, remove the mackerels from the oven then transfer to a serving dish. Serve and enjoy warm.

Strawberry Apple Chicken

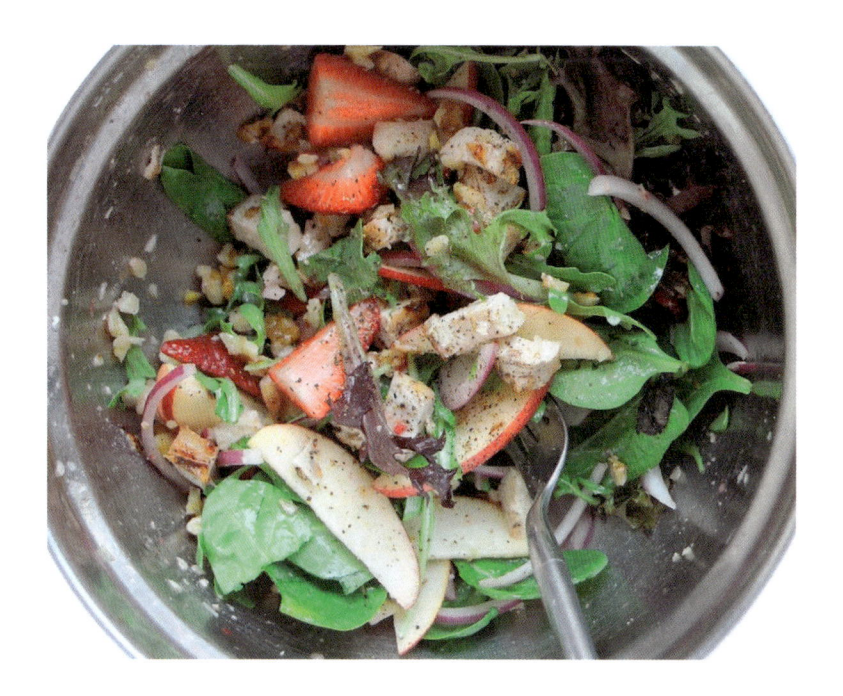

Fresh, tasteful, and healthy are three words that best describe this menu. Apple and strawberry are known for high content of antioxidants. Also, chicken is a great source of protein that you can consume moderately if you have cancer.

Serves: 4

Time: 15 mins.

Ingredients:

- ¼ cup organic chicken breast
- ½ cup sliced apple
- ¼ cup sliced strawberry
- ½ cup chopped cabbage
- 2 tablespoons olive oil
- ½ teaspoon pepper
- 1 teaspoon minced garlic
- 1-teaspoon mustard
- ½ cup water

Directions:

1. Set your skillet to preheat on medium heat then pour olive oil into it.

2. Once it is hot, stir in chicken, minced garlic, and pepper then sears until the chicken is no longer pink.

3. Remove the chicken from heat then using a fork shred the chicken.

4. Add cabbage into the skillet together with pepper and mustard then stir well.

5. Remove the skillet from heat then add sliced apple and strawberries into the skillet then mix well.

6. Transfer to a serving dish then serve immediately.

Roasted Tofu with Sesame Seeds

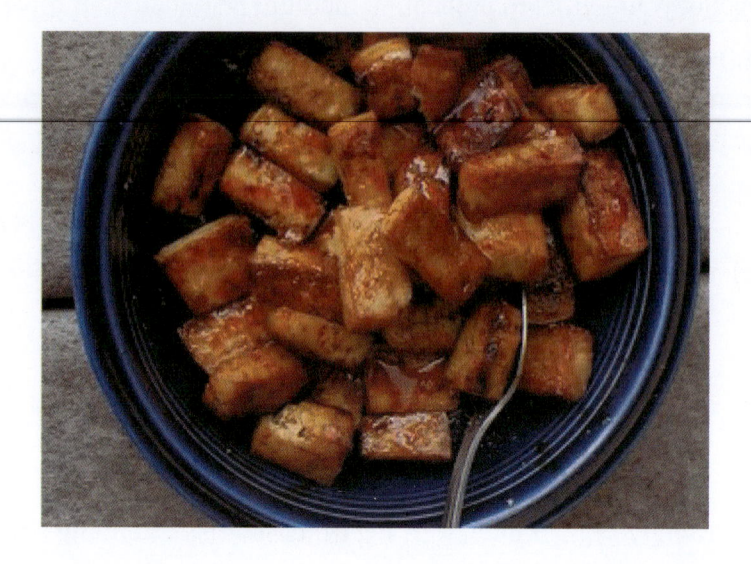

The benefits of tofu for cancer patients are without doubts. But I want to focus more on the benefits of sesame seeds for cancer treatment.

Serves: 4

Time: 15 mins.

Ingredients:

- 1 lb. firm tofu
- 1 tablespoon minced garlic
- ½ teaspoon cayenne pepper
- ½ teaspoon thyme
- ½ teaspoon pepper
- 2 teaspoons olive oil
- 2 tablespoons soy sauce
- 1-tablespoon sesame seeds

Directions:

1. Combine minced garlic with cayenne pepper, thyme, pepper, soy sauce, and olive oil. Mix well.

2. Cut the tofu into cubes then dip in the spice mixture. Set aside.

3. Preheat an oven to 400 °F then lines a baking pan with aluminum foil.

4. Spread the tofu in the prepared baking pan then drizzle the spice mixture over the tofu.

5. Bake for 12 minutes until the tofu is lightly brown.

6. Remove from the oven then transfers to a serving dish.

7. Sprinkle sesame seeds on top then serve with steamed broccoli. Enjoy!

Sautéed Carrots

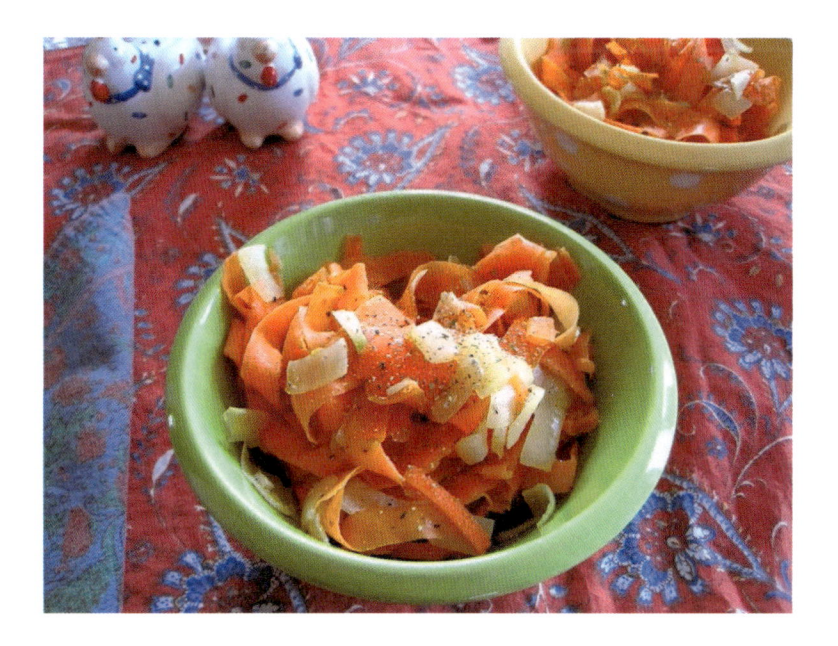

This kind of snack is easy to make and a good source of food for cancer patients. If you get bored eating the same snack over and over, you can substitute it with other kinds of sautéed veggies of fruits that are good for fighting cancer cells, such as zucchini, broccoli, cauliflower, apples, and eggplants.

Serves: 4

Time: 15 mins.

Ingredients:

- 1 lb. carrots
- 1 ½ teaspoons pepper
- 3 teaspoons butter
- 2 tablespoons raw honey

Directions:

1. Peel and cut carrots into sticks then sets aside.

2. Preheat a skillet over medium heat then add butter into it.

3. Once the butter is melted, stir in the carrot sticks then season with pepper. Cook until the carrot is wilted but still crispy.

4. Turn the stove off then quickly drizzle honey over the carrots then stir well. Transfer to a serving dish then enjoys!

Original Roasted Pumpkin

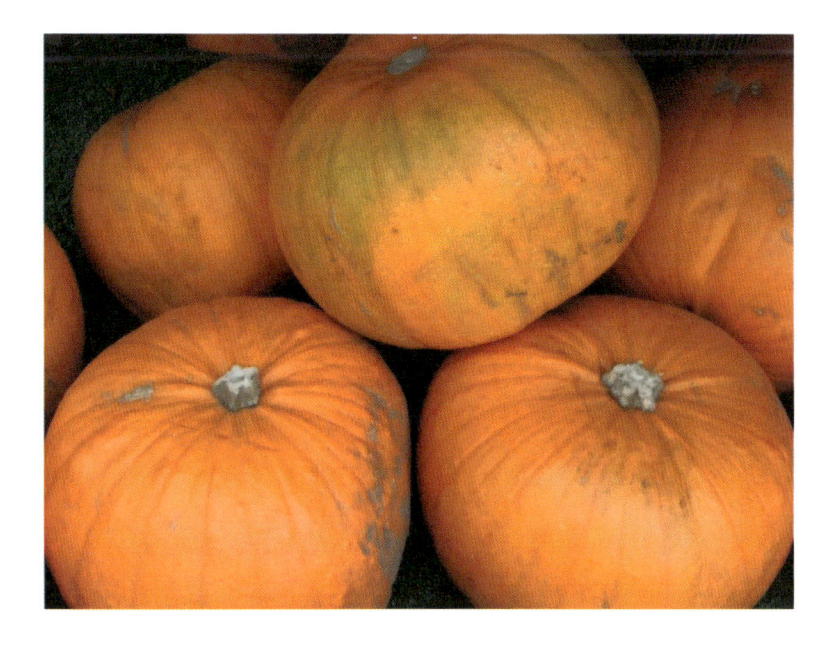

Just like other orange color fruits and vegetables, pumpkin is also rich in antioxidant from its beta-carotene content. It is proven that antioxidant is very important to not only prevent but also cure cancer. It is an agent exists in the pumpkin that naturally fights cancer cells.

Serves: 4

Time: 30 mins.

Ingredients:

- 1 lb. pumpkin
- 2 tablespoons olive oil
- 1-tablespoon mustard
- 1-teaspoon pepper

Directions:

1. Preheat an oven to 200°F then lines a baking sheet with parchment paper. Set aside.

2. Combine olive oil with mustard and pepper then mix well.

3. Peel and cut the pumpkin into wedges then rub them with the spice mixture.

4. Place the pumpkin on the prepared baking sheet then spread evenly.

5. Bake for 30 minutes until the pumpkin is tender and lightly golden.

6. Once it is done, remove from the oven then transfer to a serving dish. Serve and enjoy!

Brown Eggplant Black Pepper

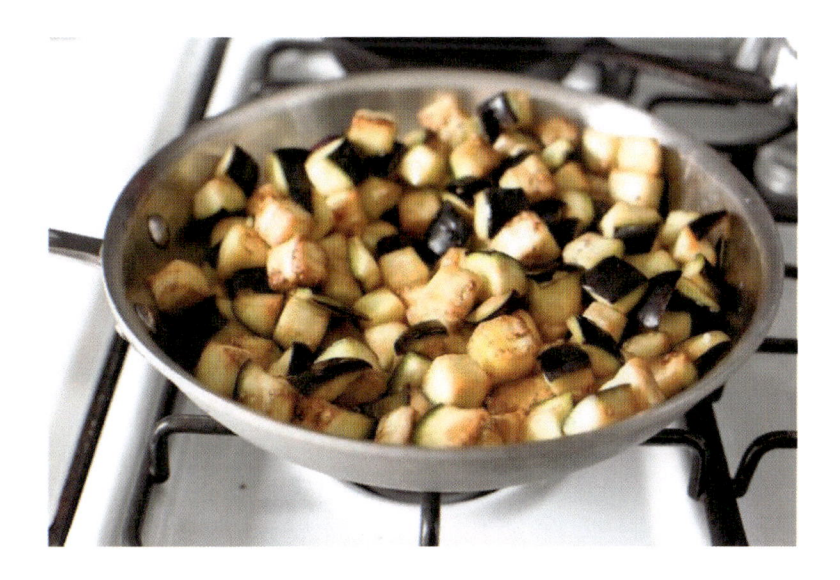

If in the previous recipe we have known the benefits of eggplants for a cancer cure, we now learn another way of cooking this veggie in its simplest way. This baked eggplant recipe is very easy to make. You can also add some broccoli and carrots in the pan to have some selections of veggies in one serving.

Serves: 2

Time: 60 mins.

Ingredients:

- 1 lb. Eggplant
- 1-tablespoon olive oil
- 2 teaspoons minced garlic
- ½ teaspoon black pepper

Directions:

1. Preheat an oven to 400 F then coats a baking sheet with cooking spray. Set aside.

2. Cut the eggplant into slices then rub with minced garlic.

3. Arrange the sliced eggplant on the prepared baking sheet then brush olive oil on them.

4. Sprinkle black pepper on top then bakes for 30 minutes.

5. Remove from the oven then flip the eggplant.

6. Bake for another 30 minutes then transfer to a serving dish. 7. Enjoy!

Green Spinach Fritter

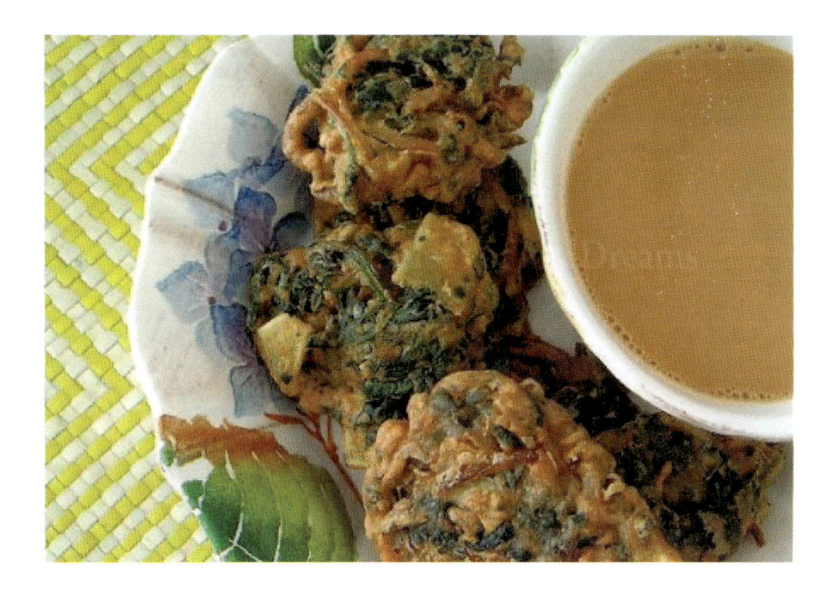

Greens fight cancer better than any other medical treatment available in this modern era. Spinach is one alternative. Eating this veggie that is full of fiber and iron is a great way to help you with your craving for food.

Serves: 4

Time: 20 mins.

Ingredients:

- 2 cups chopped spinach
- 2 tablespoons chopped onion
- ¾ cup coconut milk
- 1 cup almond flour
- ¼ cup melted butter
- 1-teaspoon garlic
- ½ teaspoon black pepper

Directions:

1. Set an oven to 350 F then line a baking sheet with parchment paper.

2. Combine all ingredients in a bowl then mix well.

3. Shape the mixture into balls forms then arrange on the prepared baking sheet.

4. Bake for 20 minutes until the spinach balls are set.

5. Remove from the oven then transfer the spinach balls to a serving dish. Serve and enjoy!

Coconut Ginger Muffins

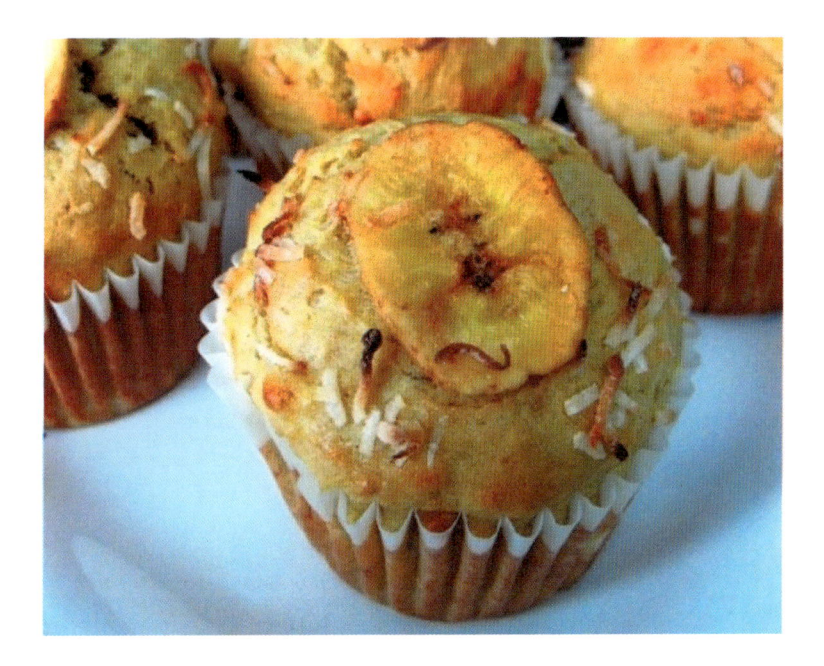

The function of ginger to cure and prevent cancer is well known. Coconut is also a good source of plant-based fat that is recommended for cancer patients. Grab one for an easy and quick meal.

Serves: 8

Time: 20 mins.

Ingredients:

- ½ cups coconut flour
- ½ cup grated coconut
- 1 ½ cups coconut milk
- ¼ cup olive oil
- 3 tablespoons raw honey

Directions:

1. Preheat an oven to 400 F then coat 8 muffin cups with cooking spray. Set aside.

2. Combine coconut flour and grated coconut in a bowl. Mix well.

3. In a separate bowl, place coconut milk, olive oil, and raw honey then stir until incorporated.

4. Pour the liquid mixture over the dry mixture then mix until combined.

5. Divide the mixture into the prepared muffin cups then bake for 20 minutes or until the top of the muffins are lightly golden.

6. Remove from the oven then serve immediately.

Conclusion

We have reached the end of the Battling Cancer Cookbook. Food has been proven to help heal and even reverse many chronic illnesses, including, but not limited to, cancer. This book was designed to assist with just that so, I hope you were able to find it not only useful but also fulfilling.

Until next time … Keep on cooking, and enjoying a long, and healthy life.

About the Author

Born in New Germantown, Pennsylvania, Stephanie Sharp received a Masters degree from Penn State in English Literature. Driven by her passion to create culinary masterpieces, she applied and was accepted to The International Culinary School of the Art Institute where she excelled in French cuisine. She has married her cooking skills with an aptitude for business by opening her own small cooking school where she teaches students of all ages.

Stephanie's talents extend to being an author as well and she has written over 400 e-books on the art of cooking and baking that include her most popular recipes.

Sharp has been fortunate enough to raise a family near her hometown in Pennsylvania where she, her husband and children live in a beautiful rustic house on an extensive piece of land. Her other passion is taking care of the furry members of her family which include 3 cats, 2 dogs and a potbelly pig named Wilbur.

Watch for more amazing books by Stephanie Sharp coming out in the next few months.

Author's Afterthoughts

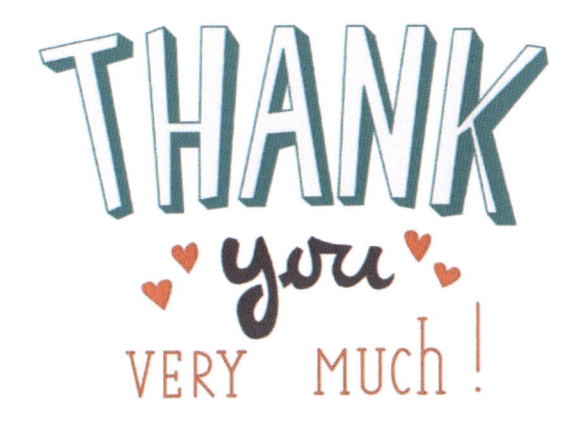

I am truly grateful to you for taking the time to read my book. I cherish all of my readers! Thanks ever so much to each of my cherished readers for investing the time to read this book!

With so many options available to you, your choice to buy my book is an honour, so my heartfelt thanks at reading it from beginning to end!

I value your feedback, so please take a moment to submit an honest and open review on Amazon so I can get valuable insight into my readers' opinions and others can benefit from your experience.

Thank you for taking the time to review!

Stephanie Sharp

For announcements about new releases, please follow my author page on Amazon.com!

You can find that at:

<https://www.amazon.com/author/stephanie-sharp>

*or Scan **QR-code** below.*

Printed in Great Britain
by Amazon